CAREER AS A

NURSE ANESTHETIST

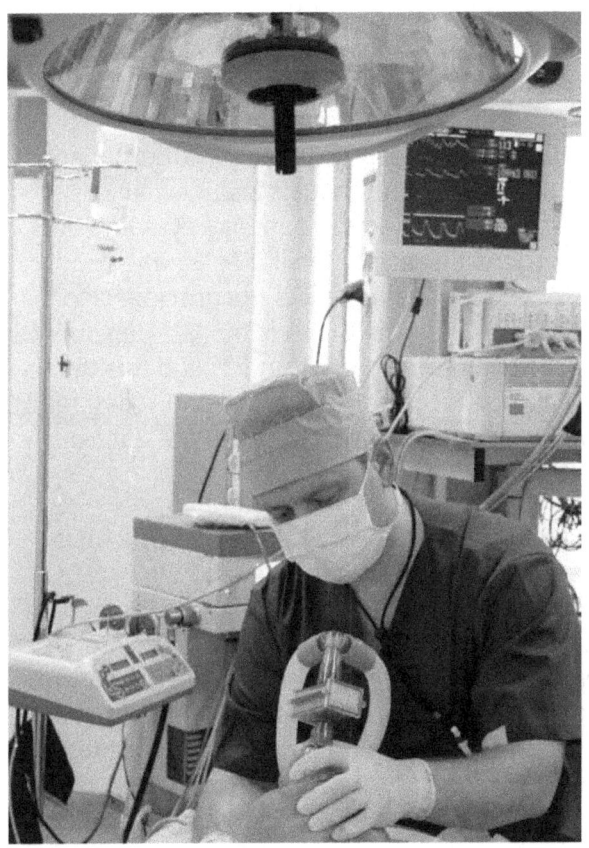

YOU'VE SEEN THE OLD WESTERN movies when someone
who has been shot is given a bullet to clench
between his teeth so he won't bite his tongue off
during surgery. Prior to the advent of anesthesia in
the mid-1800s, even the most modest of surgeries
were usually excruciatingly painful for patients. Since

then, the field of anesthesiology has advanced significantly, offering patients a painless, comfortable, and safe surgical experience.

Each year in the United States, approximately 30 million people receive anesthetics, with certified registered nurse anesthetists (CRNAs) administrating approximately 65 percent of them. The oldest recognized nursing specialists, nurse anesthetists have touched millions of lives over the years. Although anesthesia may be thought of as merely putting patients to sleep so they will not experience surgical pain, nurse anesthetists also play an important role acting as the patient's eyes and ears during surgery, essentially serving as a patient advocate because the patient is unconscious and cannot speak. Often the CRNA is the last person a patient sees before being put under, and it is the CRNA who offers comfort and confident reassurance, and then proceeds to watch over the patient like a guardian angel.

CRNAs are an integral part of the entire operative process. After inducing sleep, they monitor vital signs, adjust anesthesia levels, and wake the patient after surgery. Throughout, they are vigilant monitors of every heartbeat and every breath, as they must be ready to respond if something is not right, such as a patient having a negative response to a certain anesthetic. Fortunately, according to a recent Institute of Medicine report, due to advances in the field, anesthesia is approximately 50 times safer than it was as recently as the 1980s.

Nurse anesthetists have been blazing trails in the field since the Civil War, when they were responsible for giving soldiers ether during surgery. Since then they have been the principal providers of anesthesia care to US military personnel on the front lines. The CRNA credential was first established in 1956, and today approximately 42,000 nurse anesthetists throughout the United States administer anesthesia for all types of surgical procedures, from simple to complex. They also work in a variety of settings, from hospitals to private healthcare practices of dentists, podiatrists, ophthalmologists, plastic surgeons, and pain management specialists. On an international basis, according to the International Federation of Nurse Anesthetists, CRNAs are solely responsible for providing 60 percent of anesthesia worldwide and are the predominant providers of anesthesia in rural areas and developing countries.

Being a nurse anesthetist is exciting, challenging, and rewarding. They are among the highest paid of all nurses, with salaries typically in the six-figure range. In addition, nurse anesthetists are in great demand and have been so since the late 1980s.

If you are thinking of a career as a nurse or are currently a registered nurse (RN) who is thinking about going on to become a CRNA, this report will provide you with valuable information on everything from the history of the field and career duties, to educational requirements and a first-hand look at the field through the eyes of its practitioners.

WHAT YOU CAN DO NOW

THE FIELD OF NURSE ANESTHESIOLOGY is one of the best kept secrets of the nursing profession. You can begin right now by exploring what the field of nurse anesthesia is all about. Visit the American Association of Nurse Anesthetists (AANA) website at www.aana.com, which includes a wide range of information about the profession, from accredited educational programs to the latest news concerning this career.

If you are in high school and thinking about a career in nursing, pay special attention to your science classes, especially biology and mathematics. Volunteer in a hospital to get a feel for the overall field of nursing. Even better, talk with a nurse anesthetist about the career. You can even contact the AANA via their website and find out about opportunities to shadow a nurse anesthetist for a day so that you can have a first-hand experience of what these professionals do. Start planning for your future, write down your interests, and list your talents, strengths, and weaknesses. Your goal is to consider and ultimately determine whether or not nursing and nurse anesthesiology in particular are right for you.

If you are already a registered nurse, you can also begin preparing for a career as a nurse anesthetist. Consider your options both in terms of education and the clinical setting you would like to work in, whether it's a hospital operating room, the military, or a private practice setting. You may also want to consider the potential to specialize in fields such as plastic surgery, pediatrics, obstetrics, or cardiac care, among others. The AANA website can give you valuable information on how to apply to a certified CRNA educational program and on the board exam.

This report, which includes a history of the field, will provide much of the information you need plus resources for further research. Remember, it is never too early to start preparing for a rewarding career as a nurse anesthesiologist.

HISTORY

THE HISTORY OF THE NURSE ANESTHETIST dates back to the earliest days of medical anesthesia use in the United States. The history of anesthesiology can be traced to at least the ancient Sumerian people, who, around 4200 BC, used opium poppies as an herbal remedy. The ancient Assyrians and Egyptians also used a form of anesthesiology by putting their patients to sleep via compression of the carotid vessels in the neck. Islamic physicians became particularly adept at anesthesiology for their time, using a wide range of medicinal plants that included an anesthetic called armamentarium.

Nevertheless, the use of anesthetics remained rudimentary in terms of safety and always ensuring that the patient was anesthetized adequately. In 1799, a British chemist named Humphry Davy discovered a nitrous oxide (sometimes referred to as laughing gas) that had anesthetic effects. The discovery went unheralded until a Connecticut dentist named Horace Wells began using nitrous oxide to help patients through painful tooth surgery.

Another dentist named William Thomas Green Morton gave the first public demonstration of diethyl ether (then called sulfuric ether) as an anesthetic in Boston, on October 16, 1846. The event was so momentous that a Mr. Thomas Lee informed the city government of Boston that "I propose to erect and present to the city a monument in the form of a fountain, as an expression of gratitude for the relief of human suffering occasioned by the discovery of the anesthetic properties of sulfuric ether." The monument's construction began in 1867 and was completed on June 27, 1868.

In 1847, James Young Simpson, a Scottish obstetrician, introduced the use of chloroform, which was eventually found to have higher risks than those associated with ether. Cocaine was the first effective local anesthetic to be discovered, when it was isolated in 1859. Famed psychiatrist Sigmund Freud recommended cocaine to surgeon Carl Koller in 1884 as potentially useful in ophthalmic surgery.

Nursing became a widely recognized healthcare profession in the 1850s, largely due to the work of Florence Nightingale during the Crimean War. Nurses in the United States, such as Catherine S. Lawrence, first began to give anesthesia while caring for wounded soldiers during the Civil War. A little more than a decade after the Civil War ended, Sister Mary Bernard, a Catholic nursing sister at St Vincent's Hospital in Erie, Pennsylvania, became the first nurse known to specialize in anesthesia, providing anesthesia for the hospital surgeries.

In 1889 Alice Magaw worked as a nurse anesthetist at St Mary's Hospital in Rochester, Minnesota, later to become the world famous Mayo Clinic. Magaw was dubbed the "Mother of Anesthesia" by Dr. Charles Mayo for her numerous achievements in anesthesiology. She was particularly recognized for her expertise in the use of chloroform via the drop inhalation technique. Magaw also published her findings on the use of this technique. Titled *Observations in Anesthesia,* it is the first paper by a nurse anesthetist. In 1906, Magaw documented in an article for *Surgery, Gynecology, and Obstetrics* more than 14,000 anesthetic cases without a single complication connected to anesthesia.

A Cleveland surgeon named George Crile asked nurse Agatha Hodgins to become his anesthetist in 1908.

The following year Agnes McGee founded the first formal educational program in nurse anesthesiology at St Vincent's Hospital in Portland, Oregon. In 1914, Crile and Hodgins, who would go on to become the founder of the American Association of Nurse Anesthetists, went to France to help establish operating theatres for Allied soldiers wounded during World War I. While there, Hodgins instructed French and English physicians and nurses in techniques for administering nitrous oxide-oxygen anesthesia. After the war, Hodgins established the Lakeside Hospital School of Anesthesia, which trained nurses in anesthesia care. Her school was just one of many new programs developed after World War I, as the demand for nurse anesthetists sharply increased.

In 1931, Hodgins gathered 47 alumni of her school together in Cleveland, Ohio, to establish the AANA's precursor, the National Association of Nurse Anesthetists (NANA). The organization's first annual meeting was held in 1933 in Milwaukee, Wisconsin. Some in the medical profession, however, viewed nurse anesthetists as practicing medicine and deemed the practice illegal. In 1934, the California Supreme Court ruled that nurse anesthesiology is legal.

NANA changed its named to the American Association of Nurse Anesthetists in 1939. In 1945, the ANNA implemented a certification program, followed in 1952 by an established mechanism for accreditation. In 1956, AANA members adopted the credential of Certified Registered Nurse Anesthetist (CRNA). Over the years, numerous subspecialties in nursing anesthesiology were established, such as pediatrics and obstetrics.

No history of nurse anesthetists would be complete without paying homage to the principal anesthesia providers in combat areas in every war that the United States has been engaged. Nurse anesthetists have lost their lives and been held as prisoners of war while serving their country. They have also received many honors and decorations for their service, including the two nurse anesthetists killed in the Vietnam War whose names are engraved on the Vietnam Memorial Wall in Washington DC.

Anesthesiology has come a long way over the past century. Anesthetics are more effective and safer than ever before. Numerous anesthetic drugs are available for use in modern practice, as is a wide variety of medical equipment. Many advances have been made in the field of nurse anesthesiology as well. In 1986, for example, congress passed legislation that made nurse anesthetists the first advanced practice nursing specialists to be accorded direct reimbursement rights under the Medicare program. Despite this and other advances in the field, the US Department of Health and Human Services has indicated a growing need for additional nurse anesthetists. This need has continued as nurse anesthetists have proven to be critical and highly valued members of the surgical healthcare team.

WHERE YOU WILL WORK

THE COMBINATION OF NURSING skills and technical knowledge enables these professionals to work in every setting in which anesthesia is delivered. Employers include traditional hospital surgical suites, obstetrical delivery rooms, ambulatory surgery centers, and pain clinics, as well as the offices of physicians, plastic surgeons, ophthalmologists, dentists, and podiatrists. Nurse anesthetists also practice on a solo basis, in groups, and collaboratively. Some nurse anesthetists have independent contracting arrangements with physicians and hospitals.

A recent Practice Profile Survey conducted by AANA found that most certified registered nurse anesthetists (CRNAs) work in a hospital (35 percent) or group practice (33 percent) setting. Furthermore, almost all full-time CRNAs work primarily in one of these practice settings. The remaining CRNAs work in management, administration, and/or education.

Many nurse anesthetists work in small towns and rural settings where they manage most of the anesthesiology duties due to cost savings compared to hiring a full-time anesthesiologist (medical doctor). Nurse anesthetists also work in the US military, public health services, and Department of Veterans Affairs healthcare facilities. They may be stationed stateside or overseas, and be stationed on navy vessels and in combat zones. Overall, nurse anesthetists are the only anesthesia providers in approximately half of all hospitals and more than two-thirds of rural hospitals in the United States.

For the most part, nurse anesthetists work indoors in modern and comfortable operating rooms, clinics, and outpatient settings. These rooms are usually kept at slightly cooler temperatures. Nurse anesthetists also work in offices where they may consult with patients and conduct administrative duties. Some nurse anesthetists work in academia, where they teach future generations of nurse anesthetists, and may conduct research.

Geographically, nurse anesthetists work throughout the United States, from large metropolitan areas to smaller towns, and rural hospitals and clinics. The majority of nurse anesthetists work in general medical and surgical hospitals or physicians' offices. Other major areas of employment include nursing care facilities and home healthcare services.

Nurse anesthetists may also choose to work abroad through programs such as Health Volunteers Overseas. These positions include working in many third world countries, and involve not only anesthesia services but can also include training local hospital staff to advance their skills and knowledge of anesthesiology.

Nurse anesthetists typically have personal contracts with hospitals and physicians. According to the American Association of Nurse Anesthetists, a certified nurse anesthetist has the legal right to practice in institutional or corporate settings and can be a part of individual or group private practice.

WORK DUTIES

THE MAIN DUTY OF A NURSE ANESTHETIST is to provide patients with anesthesia during certain medical procedures, including surgery and obstetrical procedures. One of the first and most important duties is to conduct a complete assessment of patients. In assessing patients, the nurse anesthetist typically requests consultations and diagnostic studies; selects, obtains, and administers pre-anesthetic medications and fluids; and obtains informed consent from the patient or patient representative for anesthesia.

Before the patient undergoes surgery or another medical procedure, the nurse anesthetist is also responsible for providing the patient with complete knowledge of the procedure of anesthesia. This preoperative interview provides important information, such as any type of allergies a patient may have, that will help determine what type of anesthetic is appropriate, as well as overall patient care during surgery. Good communications and cooperation between the patient and the anesthesia provider are essential to ensure the safe administration of anesthesia, and to put the patient at ease concerning the administration of anesthesia. For example, instead of merely providing statistics about the safety of anesthesia that may have little meaning to patients, the nurse anesthetist may relate the risks to something that has more meaning for a patient, such as the fact that a person is about twice as likely to die in an automobile accident compared to the risk of death under anesthesia.

After going over the patient's medical history, including interpreting pre-surgical tests to determine how anesthesia will affect the patient, and interviewing the patient, the nurse anesthetist develops and implements an anesthetic plan. This includes selecting, obtaining, and administering the anesthetics, accessory drugs, and fluids (such as a blood supply), necessary to properly manage the patient under anesthetic, ensure physiologic homeostasis, and correct abnormal response to the anesthesia or surgery.

Prior to the medical procedure, the nurse anesthetist gathers all supplies and equipment necessary for caring for the patient during surgery. This includes the section of non-invasive and invasive monitoring modalities needed for gathering and interpreting a patient's physiological data. For example, depending on the specific case, the nurse anesthetist may use brain function monitors to measure the depth of anesthesia.

Once the surgery or other procedure begins, the nurse anesthetist acts as the physician's eyes and ears. After starting the patient's IV and administering a tranquilizer or mild sedative if the patient is overly nervous, the nurse anesthetist will monitor the patient's appearance and vital signs, such as heart rate, breathing rate, and blood pressure to help gauge the depth of anesthesia, and communicate to the doctor any significant changes.

During the procedure the nurse anesthetist manages a patient's airway and pulmonary status to avoid patient surgical shock, and to ensure maximum safety and comfort. Approaches to monitoring patients include the use of endotracheal intubation, mechanical ventilation, pharmacological support, respirator therapy, or extubation. The nurse is also responsible for responding to emergency situations through methods such as providing airway management, administering emergency fluids or drugs, or using cardiac life support techniques.

Following the surgery, the nurse anesthetist assists the patient with recovery from anesthesia via anesthesia reversal and extubation if necessary. The anesthetist also continues to provide other postoperative care in the post-anesthesia care unit (PACU) or, in more serious cases, such as coronary artery bypass grafting, in the critical care unit. In the PACU, the nurse anesthetist is responsible for informing the unit's staff about the patient's condition, including the type of surgery performed, the kind of anesthesia given, and estimated blood loss, as well as any complications that occurred during the surgery, such as variations in hemodynamic stability.

The nurse anesthetist may also help provide an overall assessment of the patient, including the immediate need to assess the patient's overall vital signs, airway patency (no blockage), and level of consciousness. Other assessments include level of sensation after regional anesthesia, pain status, signs of nausea and/or vomiting, patency of drainage tubes/drains, body temperature (hypothermia/hyperthermia), patency/flow rate of IV fluids, and circulation/sensation in extremities after vascular or orthopedic surgery. The amount of time a patient remains in the PACU depends on the length and type of surgery, status of regional anesthesia, and the patient's level of consciousness.

Although the majority of the anesthetists function primarily in the operating rooms of hospitals or in various medical private practices, they also provide clinical support services in other areas, such as MRI units, cardiac catheterization labs, and lithotripsy units. Services in these areas are wide ranging and include providing consultation and implementation of respiratory and ventilatory care.

The nurse anesthetist may also help manage emergency situations, and help with procedures such as cardiopulmonary resuscitation involving airway maintenance, ventilation, tracheal intubation, and management of blood, fluid, electrolyte, and acid-base balance.

In addition to their clinical duties, nurse anesthetists typically have a number of administrative responsibilities. In addition to scheduling duties, they maintain records of each anesthetic administered and record each patient's preoperative, operative, and postoperative condition. The nurse anesthetist may also prepare reports concerning other healthcare personnel, take inventories, and order supplies as well as requisition equipment and repairs. They may hold staff and committee appointments with governmental agencies, from state boards of nursing to the US Food and Drug Administration. They may also be involved in professional and standard-setting organizations, such as the American Society for Testing and Materials.

Supervisory Positions

A chief nurse anesthetist or administrative nurse anesthetist is typically the first line supervisor and has administrative responsibility for the entire anesthesia staff, especially in rural settings and in the military. At this level, the anesthetist is responsible for strategic planning, and administrative and managerial duties. The chief nurse anesthetist works with limited guidance in areas of anesthetic care. Duties include scheduling and supervising staff, students, and ancillary personnel, as well as performance evaluation and planning, organizing, directing, and controlling a program integrated with other specialties and clinics within a hospital or organization.

The chief nurse anesthetist may also serve on committees, conduct departmental reviews, and make problem-focused studies. The chief nurse keeps records to justify program goals and is also responsible for motivating personnel. Yet another administrative duty is the design and management of budget and cost-benefit analysis to ensure optimal use of resources. The chief nurse may develop protocols of anesthesia practice and provide overall leadership in applying the nursing process to patient care.

Academic Positions

Some experienced nurse anesthetists may also work in academia, typically major academic medical centers where they teach in the nurse anesthesia program and conduct clinical research. Teaching requires an understanding of different teaching styles or methods, and deciding on which method to use. Teachers also focus on providing their students with good communications skills that will allow them to communicate with both patients and other healthcare professionals. Teaching involves lesson preparation, classroom instruction, and advisory and administrative duties.

Research

As a researcher, the nurse anesthetist helps contribute to knowledge development, theory generation, and hypothesis testing in anesthesia studies. Research programs are broad based and may include both basic laboratory work and a focused clinical research program. Research may involve experimental design of projects, including the design and organization of clinical trials and statistical analyses.

Researchers are required to communicate and function across disciplines and use advanced research methodologies and technology. They also are required to communicate research findings both to the scientific and social policy communities, and they may be called upon to relate research to the development and implementation of healthcare policy, both locally and nationally.

The nurse anesthetist researcher may help draft proposals and other requests for research funding, as well as contribute to books, scientific journals, and other publications. These nurses write for publications such as *Nurse Anesthesia, Anesthesiology, Journal of the American Medical Association (JAMA)*, and *Nursing Research*. They may present research studies and findings at professional meetings and symposiums on a national and international basis.

NURSE ANESTHETISTS TELL THEIR OWN STORIES

I Am a CRNA

"I had always wanted to be a nurse but, when I started nursing school, I intended to work as an RN in a hospital, doing what I considered to be typical nursing duties and following doctors' orders. However, during a clinical rotation in my senior year, I ended up in the OR observing a routine operation. When the other students and I walked into the OR, the nurse anesthetist was just beginning to set up for the case.

I began observing him arranging and checking the equipment, and soon found myself watching him throughout the operation. I was impressed by his professionalism and with the responsibilities he seemed to have. He appeared to work as part of the surgical team, but also in a very independent way that didn't require constant physician supervision. When I recapped my experience to my professor, my enthusiasm was so great that she suggested I look into nurse anesthesia, something I had never heard of just a few days earlier.

Because of my own lack of knowledge about nurse anesthesia, I wasn't surprised that my friends and family were wondering what my new career choice was all about. I still get a similar reaction today when I tell people what I do for a living. I now use these moments as opportunities to educate the public about nurse anesthetists and their important work and impact in the field of healthcare.

I've never regretted my decision to become a nurse anesthetist. The job comes with incredible responsibility, and it is very rewarding when I deliver a patient safely into the capable hands of the recovery rooms staff. My job is to put patients to sleep safely and make sure they have a comfortable operating experience. Though emergencies in anesthesia are rare, they do happen, and I'm proud of the fact that I'm counted on to recognize and resolve any problems. Each time we roll the patient into the recovery room, I feel as though I have just helped to achieve a great victory for the patient.

There are stresses to the job, at least for me. In the hospital where I work, we do not have shifts. Instead, each day we work until all the cases are finished. I'm also not a big fan of being on-call, but I find my profession to be very fulfilling. Nurse anesthetists have an incredible responsibility to provide vigilant patient care every day. We also serve the patients by protecting and advocating for patients during their most vulnerable moments."

I Started My Own Business

"I had been a practicing RN for several years and was ready to make a change in my career. I wanted more autonomy in my work, and I wanted to take a step up in my education. I knew a nurse anesthetist at the hospital where I worked in the ER, and she assured me that in her many years working in nursing she had more independence than in any other position she ever held.   When she told me that some nurse anesthetists work as independent and autonomous practitioners, who essentially have a private practice and perform their duties without the need for physician involvement, I was intrigued.

I was already married and had two children, which meant I had to consider carefully the decision to return to school, considering both the time and money involved. I talked it over with my husband and my kids, and we decided as a family that, if that was what I wanted, we could all make it work.

The hardest thing about returning to school was that I went from being an expert in my current field, emergency medicine, to just another student. Of course, my work background had given me a strong foundation in nursing and healthcare, which made school much easier. I also found the clinical experience in school much less daunting than when I was an undergraduate, since I had already worked with too many patients to count.

After graduation, I took a job with an independent anesthesia group for a year and then decided to start my own business. The toughest part of starting the business was finding the money to purchase the necessary equipment. In the beginning, I was the owner and sole employee, but eventually I built the business up so that I now have 20 employees, counting the non-clinical staff.

Although I loved my clinical duties as a nurse anesthetist, I now work solely in an administrative role, overseeing nurse anesthetist staffing for our clients, which include several hospitals and private practices. Part of the reason for this move to a desk job was that it enables me to spend more time with my family.

Do I miss clinical work? I do, but I'm finding my new role to be very rewarding. I don't like working with the ins-and-outs of the health insurance industry. I do enjoy being able to spend more time with my staff, and knowing that I'm helping to provide top-notch services to many patients."

I Work in the Military

"I am a military trained CRNA and work full time as an Army CRNA. The scope of my practice in the military enables me to independently administer every type of anesthetic to every type of patient. I served on the front lines in Iraq and was privileged to provide services to wounded soldiers. I escorted critically wounded patients in ground ambulances, C-130 transport planes, and Black Hawks helicopters. During these trips, I placed central venous access lines, provided pain relief via regional anesthetic blocks, and secured burned air passages.

When I returned to the states and was assigned a post, I found myself practicing primarily in vascular and open heart surgeries. I went on to become, for a brief time, a chief CRNA at an Army community hospital that had lost its anesthesiologist. I now work in an Army medical center as a staff CRNA, and I am also an adjunct faculty member in the Army Nurse Anesthesia program, where our primary goal is to train people as nurse anesthetists who will be deployed during wars, civil disorders, natural disasters, and other humanitarian missions.

I oversee five to 15 student registered nurse anesthetists at any one time, and I have a good one-on-one relationship with all my students. I firmly believe that some of the finest nurse anesthetists are trained by the military. I'm proud of our work in the program, which trains CRNAs to work in some of the most difficult circumstances.

I'm a military man through and through, but I don't think the military is for everyone. One of the reasons I became a nurse anesthetist was that I wanted to practice independently. Independent practice for nurse anesthetists has long been the norm in the military, partly because of the fact that there are not enough anesthesiologists (doctors) to staff every deployed location where anesthesia services are needed. Nevertheless, in the military, you have to be able to take and follow orders that go beyond the operating room.

I highly recommend a career as a nurse anesthetist. Although I have not worked as a civilian, I know many ex-colleagues who have returned to civilian life and thoroughly enjoy working as a nurse anesthetist in the civilian sector. Personally, what I like about being a nurse anesthetist is that I get to work with one patient at a time. It can sometimes be stressful for patients undergoing surgery, even hardened military men. I feel it is my duty not only to provide anesthesia care but to help them through the process and take away some of their anxiousness."

I Am a CRNA Student

"I had considered going to medical school but ultimately chose a CRNA program to become a nurse anesthetist. I had been interested in medical anesthesiology, but I liked what I heard about the autonomy that nurse anesthetists have. In the end, a major factor in my decision was that I could become a practicing nurse anesthetist much faster and for less money than attending medical school to become an anesthesiologist, which not only required four years of medical school, but also a medical residency which could take three more years, and then a couple more years for an anesthesia fellowship. I would also be lying if I didn't say that the six figure salary in the nursing job is also attractive.

I first earned my bachelor's degree and RN, and then worked for two years in a cardiovascular/surgical ICU (intensive care unit) before returning to school. I have to say, I thought CRNA school would be easy. I guess I was comparing it to medical school and considering the fact that I had a few years of clinical experience under my belt. But it's definitely the hardest thing I've ever done in an academic sense. Essentially, the program is cramming the equivalent of two years of medical school into one year.

My program first features classroom work and then the clinical experience. I quickly found that you have a very short time to learn an overwhelming amount of information, which you have to know backwards and forwards. In fact, you have to know it as well as anesthesiologists who are MDs. As a result, the CRNA program is intense.

Recently, I had three midterms in one day and was up studying all night for a week. Initially, I had trouble dealing with the stress of school, but I decided to do some research after I dropped 20 pounds because I wasn't eating. I learned how to compartmentalize my workload and handle each task on a priority basis. I learned that I could physiologically calm myself with deep breathing and other relaxation techniques. The point is, get ready to be challenged and make sure you learn how to deal with it.

I'm not trying to make school sound too scary, though. I really enjoy it for the most part. I like science and nursing and people, and I've made new friends, which is good because some of my other friends have a hard time understanding how busy I am.

Right now, I'm getting a little nervous for clinicals but I'm already preparing for my OR experience. I have had my orientation at the hospital, and I am going back to meet my preceptors and learn how to do a machine check.

If I had any advice for high school students

thinking about a career in this field, I can only say do everything you can to prepare for college and the rigors of a CRNA program. Develop good study and time management habits as early as you can."

PERSONAL QUALIFICATIONS

IN ADDITION TO A FORMAL EDUCATION in the science and practice of anesthesiology, the nurse anesthetist should possess a number of personal attributes and qualities that benefit job performance. As with all healthcare workers, the nurse anesthetist should be a compassionate and patient advocate. At times, the nurse anesthetist has the best up-to-the minute patient data and information which may be vital to a medical procedure's outcome. In some cases, because the patient is under an anesthetic, the anesthetist must ensure that the patient is not placed in a dangerous position that could lead to injury or worse.

Nurse anesthetists are totally dedicated to the well-being of their patients, as they often care for them in situations that can result in negative patient outcomes, and sometimes even death. As a result, they are constantly vigilant, realizing that a patient's status can change drastically at any time.

They should also have critical thinking skills, be able to observe accurately and make decisions accordingly. The ability to think quickly and decisively is important as the nurse anesthetist may be required to formulate a care plan on the spot and have a good rationale for picking a particular course of action. These nurses thrive on challenges and have a high level of self-confidence. They must have faith in their ability to make the right decision and do what needs to be done, especially because the nurse is often faced with situations where second or third opinions are not readily available.

Organization is also a quality you must have. In the clinical setting, you will be responsible for a multitude of tasks involved in administering an anesthetic and monitoring the patient. It is essential to have everything organized, from the proper medications and equipment to emergency contingencies. Organization is also invaluable on the administrative side of nursing.

Determination is another good quality for anyone seeking to become a nurse anesthetist. This quality is needed to complete the demanding training needed to qualify as a nurse anesthetist. The ability to focus will also help you in your studies, as well as on the job.

Because of the intense nature of the work, the nurse anesthetist must be emotionally stable. Nurse anesthetists work with all kinds of patients, from young to old, from those with relatively stable conditions to those in life-threatening situations. Surgeries can develop into stressful situations, especially when something goes wrong, and sometimes patients die. The nurse anesthetist must be able to handle these situations. In addition, nurse anesthetists work with a wide range of healthcare professionals, from surgeons to anesthesiologists to other nurses. As a result, they must be able to work well as part of a team.

The good news about personal qualities is that they can be cultivated. Perhaps you feel you aren't as patient as you could be and that this might hinder your performance on the job. Or you may fear that you might not have the determination to make it through the years of schooling necessary to become a nurse anesthetist. First of all, congratulate yourself on recognizing areas for improvement, and then set out to practice the qualities you would like to improve.

ATTRACTIVE FEATURES

WORKING AS A NURSE ANESTHETIST has numerous advantages. First, they are in great demand nationwide, meaning that job opportunities are excellent. As a result, the career offers job security. The need for these professionals will actually increase in years to come as baby boomers reach retirement age, and people live longer than they used to. In addition, nurse anesthetists also have a competitive advantage over physician anesthesiologists considering costs to the government and society. The advantage lies in the fact that approximately eight nurse anesthetists can be educated for the cost of one physician anesthesiologist.

The most obvious attractive feature of being a nurse anesthetist is that it offers a great deal of personal satisfaction. Nurse anesthetists help make a significant difference in peoples' lives. While their interaction with patients may be relatively brief, the time they do spend with them can help them through an often extremely stressful situation. Many nurse anesthetists believe that the ability to make the anesthesia and surgical experience easier is one of the most rewarding aspects of their job.

Being a nurse anesthetist also offers job flexibility in

terms of work environments, which may include hospitals, private doctors' offices, government agencies, and the military. The nurse anesthetist has the opportunity to choose to work in a subspecialty, such as cardiac care, critical care, or ambulatory anesthesia.

Being a nurse anesthetist is never boring, as the job includes daily challenges of dealing with new patients and illnesses. Furthermore, the science of medicine and anesthesiology is constantly evolving.

Interaction with patients is often one-on-one, providing a more personal aspect to the work. Although nurse anesthetists, especially those who work in large metropolitan hospitals, are often supervised by physicians, they also enjoy a great deal of autonomy and work more independently than any other advanced practice nurse.

Because of the shortage of nurse anesthetists, opportunities exist for nurse anesthetists to provide their services in ways other than as full-time employees. Some nurse anesthetists no longer have a primary employer but contract out their services to different hospitals and organizations as needed.

Professional respect is another advantage. Nurses of all types typically earn the respect of patients and families since they play a key role in the patient's comfort during the surgical experience. Nurse anesthetists also have the respect of their colleagues as vital members of the healthcare team.

Nurse anesthetists are among the highest paid specialists within nursing, typically making over six figures a year, a salary that is often double that of a registered nurse (RN). In addition, the job includes good benefits, and the current shortage of nurse

anesthetists means that many employers offer
signing bonuses.

UNATTRACTIVE FEATURES

ACCORDING TO A RECENT STUDY, one of the primary
negative issues is the stress that comes with the job.
Occupational-related stressors are connected to
patient care, anesthesia work in general,
interpersonal job relationships, inadequate surgical
preparation, the operating room environment itself,
and various physical stress factors in a job that can
sometimes require a nurse anesthetist to be in the
operating room for many hours. Nurse anesthetists
are so dedicated to their professional duties,
patients, and colleagues, that they often do not take
vacation time or sick leave.

The good news is that CRNAs report that they find
numerous coping mechanisms to handle their job's
stress. For example, in dealing with operating room
stressors, CRNAs focus intently upon the task at hand
enabling them to block out other issues. CRNAs also
use humor on the job and find interesting hobbies to
take their mind off of work at the end of the day.

Another factor to consider when planning a career in
almost any area of nursing is the potential exposure
to viruses, bacteria, chemicals, and other harmful
substances within the hospital environment. Nurse
anesthetists seldom work a regular 9-to-5 schedule.
They are likely to work various shifts, including
weekends, and often work overtime when required.
You may also be on call, meaning that no matter
what, late night or a holiday, you must go to the
hospital for surgery when you are needed. Nurses

working in rural areas and small towns are likely to be on call more due to the limited number of physicians or other nurse anesthetists working in their clinic or hospital.

Something which may be considered a negative largely depends on your outlook concerning the extensive education and training for the career. Graduate courses in anesthesiology are intense and often push students to new levels of achievement. Furthermore, the time needed to earn certification as a CRNA may increase in coming years when CRNA schools end their master's degree programs in nurse anesthetics in favor of the Doctor of Nursing Practice (DNP) degree. Some may view the education requirements to become a nurse anesthetist as a burden while others see it as a challenge that they willingly accept, knowing that more intense training increases their ability to function in the operating room at the highest level possible.

Another issue that a person interested in a career as a nurse anesthetist should consider is liability insurance. Although nurse anesthetists make an excellent salary, most are required to obtain liability, or malpractice insurance, and can pay anywhere from $1,500 to $10,000 a year for such insurance. Furthermore, if a nurse anesthetist is named in a lawsuit, the costs can go up. Fortunately, malpractice insurance is sometimes paid for in whole or in part by the employer. Nevertheless, many nurse anesthetists carry their own insurance as independent contractors, or additional insurance to that supplied by the employer.

EDUCATION AND TRAINING

CERTIFIED REGISTERED NURSE Anesthetists (CRNAs) are among the most advanced and highest paid nurses because of their expertise and responsibilities, especially within the field of surgery. Their knowledge is both broad and specialized, enabling them to work in a technical, fast-paced, and demanding environment. As a result, the educational requirements to become certified in this advanced nursing specialty require an undergraduate degree, at least a year's experience as a practicing registered nurse (RN) in an acute care setting, and then a graduate degree from a certified CRNA college program.

Most nurse anesthetists begin their educational careers by obtaining a Bachelor of Science in Nursing degree (BSN). These are typically four year programs focusing on the science and principles of nursing. The first two years feature primarily pre-nursing courses in the humanities, and the social and natural sciences. The goal is to provide students with a more complete understanding of the world, and basic science education in anatomy and physiology, biology, chemistry, and nutrition. Another important goal is to develop good communications skills, which requires taking English writing courses.

The final two years feature courses in nursing and medicine. These may include health assessment, principles and application of nursing interventions, information technology, and public health. Courses also focus on specific patient populations, such as pediatric, adult, and geriatric nursing.

To become a registered nurse (RN), only two years of training are required. Although most RNs earn the full undergraduate BSN degree, it is possible to graduate from a two-year associate degree program. For those RNs with an associate degree, as well as others who may have a bachelor's degree in a non-nursing field, many nurse anesthetist programs offer accelerated BSN programs that can require anywhere from one to two years. For working RNs, these programs are sometimes offered in a flexible format to allow the student to continue working.

CRNA Training

There are over 100 accredited nurse anesthesia programs that use more than 1,700 approved clinical sites. The programs must be accredited by the Council on Accreditation of Nurse Anesthesia Programs, which publishes a list of accredited nurse anesthesia educational programs annually. The list is available on the American Association of Nurse Anesthetists (AANA) Web site.

CRNA programs typically range from two- to three-years in length and include clinical training within community and university-based hospitals. Despite the number of CRNA programs, competition is high as there are still not enough programs to meet the growing demand for nurse anesthetists. As a result, these programs typically look for RNs with ICU (intensive care unit) nursing experience and a high GPA. However, even if the GPA is not especially high, an applicant still can be accepted into a program by demonstrating maturity, retaking core courses, and demonstrating an ability to handle graduate work.

In addition to nursing courses, there are courses in areas such as anatomy, physiology, chemistry, biochemistry, microbiology, pharmacology, psychology, and other behavioral sciences. There are also courses in the principles of anesthesia practice. These courses include instructions in physics, pain management, and medical technology and equipment. For those students considering a career in academia and research, courses may also focus on statistics and methods of scientific inquiry. Some include a chance to participate in faculty research.

All CRNA programs also include supervised clinical experience in hospital departments such as surgery, maternity, pediatrics, and psychiatry, as well as in ambulatory clinics, nursing care facilities, public health departments, and home health agencies. The clinical component is designed to give students hands-on clinical experience to further their education in anesthesia techniques, theory, and overall patient care. Depending on the particular program, the student graduates with either a master's or a doctoral degree in nursing, allied health, or biological and clinical sciences. Nurse anesthesia students receive a median of 1,651 hours of clinical experience.

Upon graduation, the graduate must take a certification examination through the National Board on Certification and Recertification of Nurse Anesthetists (NBCRNA). In order to take the examination, a transcript is necessary to show that the graduate has completed 705 contact hours in anesthesia. In addition CRNAs must continue their education throughout their career via continuing education classes. CRNAs must seek recertification every two years. The recertification process reviews CRNA qualifications in several areas, including current licensure as a registered nurse and continued education credits.

EARNINGS

A CAREER AS A NURSE ANESTHETIST is one of the highest paying careers in the field of nursing. In 1999, the national average salary for CRNAs was about $102,000, the first time that the average salary for this profession reached the six-figure mark. By 2006, the average annual salary had jumped to $140,000, and by 2009 had reached $157,724 a year, as reported by the AMGA Medical Group Compensation and Financial Survey. According to a 2009 CNNMoney Web site survey, the top salary as a nurse anesthetist was $214,000 a year. In 2010, the average annual salary for a nurse anesthetist was $166,000 a year, with the top 10 percent of CRNAs earning $175,000 a year or more.

According to national salary data updated in May 2011, the average salary for a nurse anesthetist ranged from $79,313 to $163,463 dollars a year. When counting in bonuses and profit sharing, the average salary range reached $183,446. The top paying metropolitan areas for this occupation include the California cities of Oakland, San Francisco, and San Jose, as well as New York City and Baltimore.

Nurse anesthetists' salaries are also dependent on the setting. Operating room nurse anesthetists make significantly more money that those working for international organizations such as the World Health Organization and Peace Corps, where they make only marginally better salaries than their general nursing counterparts. While a nurse anesthetist working in a hospital can expect a median annual salary of

$155,000 a year, the WHO and Peace Corps workers generally make about $50,000 a year. Although this is quite a reduction in income, most of these workers will rightly point out that they are not doing it for the money.

Even when it comes to the low end of the salary range, which is typically where less experienced practitioners start, nurse anesthetist salaries are extremely attractive. Survey data also show that salaries typically rise as the nurse anesthetist gains experience. For example, a recent survey found that the highest average salaries were held by those nurse anesthetists who had 20 years of experience.

Benefit packages for nurse anesthetists are also inviting. In addition to salary, CRNAs receive paid vacation, professional liability insurance, and sick time. They also receive medical, life, and dental insurance. Some institutions pay for them to attend professional meetings and have allowances for further schooling, as well as tuition assistance for family members, especially in the case of academic institutions. Pension plans are also common, often with the employer making contributions to the plan.

OPPORTUNITIES

CERTIFIED REGISTERED NURSE ANESTHETISTS (CRNAs) are in high demand and have numerous opportunities for general or specialty practice throughout the United States. According to one preliminary study, over 50 percent of hospitals have openings for CRNAs. Overall, nurse anesthetists are one of the top 10 recruited healthcare specialties.

The rising number of healthcare procedures requiring anesthesia has helped lead to an increased need for CRNAs, as has the number of currently practicing nurse anesthetists who are retiring. Other factors include a growing elderly population, the rising median age of nurse anesthetists, and technological advances. As a result, the number of nurse anesthetist jobs is increasing very fast.

Job opportunities for nurse anesthetists are expected to vary by employment setting. For example, employment in the field is expected to grow more slowly in hospitals, but rapid growth is expected in outpatient facilities.

The need for all types of nurses, including nurse anesthetists, is so great that a recent Institute of Medicine report recommended that colleges and universities increase the number of nurses graduating with bachelor's degrees by at least 50 percent within the coming decade. The report also recommended that nurses with associate degrees and diplomas should be encouraged to enter bachelor's degree programs within five years of graduation.

A major move is underway for CRNA programs to abandon their master's degree programs and implement doctoral programs for training nurse anesthetists. While a doctoral program would in most cases require more time and be more intensive, the AANA has noted several advantages to earning a doctorate instead of a master's. Not only would the change increase knowledge and expertise in the practice, but it would also provide parity with other clinical practitioners, such as physical therapists and speech pathologists.

Numerous studies and surveys have made findings

that bode well for the future of nurse anesthetists as an independent field within healthcare. A study published in Health Affairs, examined approximately 500,000 cases in 14 states that had removed the federal physician supervision requirement for nurse anesthetists. The study found that outcomes did not differ between these states and the states that require physician supervision over nurse anesthetists. The study also established that patient outcomes are no different whether anesthesia services are provided by physician anesthesiologists, CRNAs, or CRNAs supervised by physicians. Another study published in the Journal of Nursing Economics, found that CRNAs acting as the sole anesthesia provider cost 25 percent less than the next lowest cost model. Overall, the increased training and trend towards independence from physician supervision mean even more opportunities for the nurse anesthetist.

The field also provides numerous opportunities for new challenges and advancements. For example, nurse anesthetists can consider teaching or administrative positions, and involvement in research. Some nurse anesthetists also acquire other advanced-practice nursing qualifications, which enable them to be involved in a wider range of nursing activities.

There are also opportunities to start your own business providing nurse anesthetist services as an independent contractor. Some of these independent contractors have grown from sole ownership enterprises to employing numerous nurse anesthetists and other staff.

GETTING STARTED

IF YOU'VE DECIDED THAT THE CHALLENGING and rewarding career of a nurse anesthetist may be right for you, you can get started now on working toward your goal. If you are still in high school, you can start by taking the most challenging college preparation courses your school offers. However, do not ignore your other classes because colleges consider a student's overall GPA. If you are already working as a registered nurse, you should gear your on-the-job experiences toward acute care, which is typically the kind of experience nurse anesthesia degree programs require.

There is no time like the present to start thinking about your school choices. High school students should first focus on their undergraduate education. Investigate Bachelor of Science in Nursing (BSN) programs at different colleges, considering factors such as each nursing school's overall reputation and the ability of students to gain real-world experience in acute care. When it is time to enter a master's program, thoroughly research schools, including checking the reputation of the academic nursing program. Remember, your goal is to choose a school that best fits your professional interests and goals. For example, if you think you might like to specialize in pediatric anesthesiology, look for a school with a strong reputation in this area.

A recommendation for anyone considering the career is to find a practicing CRNA to shadow for a day or two. For working nurses, this may be as easy as asking to shadow a colleague. For those not yet in a healthcare profession, your local hospital, outpatient surgery clinic, or nursing program may be able to help find a nurse anesthetist for you to shadow. Shadowing will not only provide you with a first-hand look at what these professionals do, but will also provide important information about the profession so that you can demonstrate a solid grasp of the field during the application process.

The cost of higher education has increased dramatically, so this is also a good time to start looking for ways to pay for college and subsequent graduate school. If you are a high school student, talk to your guidance counselor at school for information on obtaining financial help to attend college. Working nurses can look into various loan programs, including loan repayment programs offered by the military and the Indian Health Service. For example, nursing professionals serving on the US Army Reserve Health Care team may be eligible for up to $50,000 toward repaying nursing school loans.

Scholarships and grants are also available, especially for an undergraduate education. Two good sites for various scholarship opportunities are the American Association of Colleges of Nurses at http://www.aacn.nche.edu /Education/financialaid.htm and the Nurses for a Healthier Tomorrow website at http://www.nursesource.org /education_info.html. The good news for working nurses is that some hospitals and anesthesia groups will help cover tuition. It is important to remember that the cost of graduate school may be as high as $25,000 or more, but that the return on investment is well worth it considering the pay scale for nurse anesthetists.

ASSOCIATIONS

American Association of Critical Care Nurses
http://www.aacn.org

American Association of Nurse Anesthetists
http://www.aana.com

American Nurses Association
http://www.nursingworld.org

American Society of PeriAnesthesia Nurses
http://www.aspan.org

International Anesthesia Research Society
http://www.iars.org/home/default.asp

International Federation of Nurse Anesthetists
http://ifna-int.org/ifna/news.php

PERIODICALS

AANA Journal and News Bulletin
www.aana.com/Resources.aspx?id=5324

Anesthesiology Clinics of North America

Anesthesiology Review

International Student Journal of Nurse Anesthesia
www.aana.com/forstudents.aspx

Journal of Anesthesia

PeriAnesthesia Nurses Obstetric Anesthesia Digest

WEBSITES

All Nursing School
http://www.allnursingschools.com
Provides comprehensive information on
nursing education and careers

Nurse Anesthesia Forum
http://www.nurse-anesthesia.org/forum.php
A forum for nurse anesthetists to discuss a
wide range of topics in the field

Nurse Anesthetist
http://nurseanesthetist.org
Provides information on what it is like to
become a nurse anesthetist and events that
shape the professional and personal lives of
people in the profession. Includes a Web
blog section for students and practitioners